# POLYPHENOL POWER!

Polyphenols in fruit and vegetables to prevent and cure:

- Heart Disease
- Cancer
- Type 2 Diabetes
- Alzheimer's and more!

Terry Lemerond

The purpose of this book is to educate. It is not intended to serve as a replacement for professional medical advice. Any use of the information in this book is at the reader's discretion. This book is sold with the understanding that neither the publisher nor the author has any liability or responsibility for any injury caused or alleged to be caused directly or indirectly by the information contained in this book. While every effort has been made to ensure its accuracy, the book's contents should not be construed as medical advice. To obtain medical advice on your individual health needs, please consult a qualified health care practitioner.



www.TTNPublishing.com



Library of Congress Control Number: 2022906784

Print ISBN: 978-1-952507-27-4
eBook ISBN: 978-1-952507-28-1

Editor: Michele Olson
Design: Michelle LeClair
Formatting: Alt 19 Creative

Printed in the United States of America

***This book is dedicated to all the true health seekers in the world.***

# Contents

## CHAPTER 1
# Eat the Rainbow

Do you love colorful foods? Are grapes, carrots, tomatoes, broccoli, cherries, cantaloupe, and all the colors of the rainbow, not to speak of nutritional powerhouses like coffee, garlic, tea, and dark chocolate, a regular part of your diet? If so, welcome to the idea of eating for long life! If not, I hope this book will convince you of the value of a diet rich with all of the brilliant colors and natural life enhancers Mother Nature provides.

Maybe you haven't heard of the word "polyphenol" before. It's a blanket term for any of the 8,000 super healthy nutrients found in fruits, vegetables, herbs and bee products. Maybe words like flavonoids, catechins, anthocyanins, lignans, quercetin, curcuminoids, resveratrol, ellagic acid, and phenolic acids are a bit daunting. I'm sure that you've all heard of caffeine, another important polyphenol. These are all in the family of polyphenols that give fruits, vegetables, flowering herbs and spices their glowing colors and serve as natural antibiotics, insecticides, and cellular protectors for the plant world.

Not surprisingly, the polyphenols are also potent and natural protectors of human health. Since the human body cannot synthesize or store polyphenols, we rely on continuous replenishment by daily diet.

Polyphenols are so important because of their supercharged antioxidant and anti-inflammatory properties.

Let's pause a moment to look at each of their functions and how they work.

What is an antioxidant? Cut an apple and within a few minutes it will begin to turn brown due to its exposure to oxygen. We call this "rusting." Squeeze a wedge of lemon on that apple right after you cut it and it won't turn brown. The lemon is an antioxidant—it neutralizes the rusting caused by oxygen exposure.

Antioxidants neutralize disease-causing, free radical oxygen molecules, preventing them from causing the diseases caused by aging, poor lifestyle choices or unavoidable environmental factors like air pollution and toxic water.

Bear with me now.

While we need to breathe oxygen to stay alive, oxygen in our cells works just as destructively as it does on that plain apple. Your lifestyle choices and your exposure to environmental toxins over a lifetime causes "rust" (actually the correct terminology is free radical oxygen molecules) that accumulates in your cells. That free radical oxygen exposure triggers chronic inflammation, opening the door to cell aging and genetic deterioration, as well as to the diseases of aging, including cancer, heart disease, diabetes, Alzheimer's, and more.

At least 90% of all of our modern-day diseases are caused by oxidative stress and inflammation.

Wouldn't it be great if we could just squeeze lemon juice into every cell of our bodies? But seriously, there is something else we can do.

Polyphenols are also potent anti-inflammatories. For now, it's important to understand that inflammation is an underlying cause of most chronic diseases.

Polyphenols are also credited with preventing wild cellular division like is found in cancer and with preserving brain function by prevention of the deterioration of brain cells.

Most of us know someone who has high blood pressure, heart disease, cancer, arthritis, diabetes, osteoporosis, Alzheimer's disease or dementia, allergies, or asthma. Maybe you have one or more of these maladies yourself. Polyphenols are the key to preventing these chronic diseases of aging, and to promote a healthy, long life.

Seven of the top 10 leading causes of death in the United States are from chronic diseases. A diet rich in fruits and vegetables can help reduce the risk of many leading causes of illness and death, including heart disease, type 2 diabetes, some cancers and obesity.

I like to think of polyphenols as nature's perfect insurance policy. Pivotal research from the University of Barcelona in Spain confirmed that people over 65 whose diets contained at least 650 mg. of polyphenols a day were 30% less likely to die of any cause over the 12 years of the study.

Yes, we all eat veggies and fruit, right? No, catsup and French fries don't count.

But how many healthy polyphenols do you really eat? The US Centers for Disease Control and Prevention says that only one in ten of us get the recommended 1 ½ to 2 cups of fruit per day and 2 to 3 cups of vegetables. That adds up to nine servings daily, far above the recommended Five A Day that many of us grew up with.

Experts agree we need 1,000 mg of polyphenols daily to attain optimum health, especially over the age of 50. It's not easy to meet that target.

Stay with me—I'll get to the concept of supplementation in Chapter 2. But for now, let's just look at what it would take to get 1,000 mg of polyphenols a day through food alone.

Some of the highest polyphenol content is found in spices, but it is not realistic to expect you might eat four ounces of cloves in a day to get 15,000 mg of polyphenols, or four ounces of rosemary to get 1,000 mg.

It's probably also unrealistic to expect you to eat these foods to get that crucial 1,000 mg:

7.3 bowls of spinach salad

or

11 cups of green tea

or

6 red onions

or

20 bowls of cooked broccoli

We'll talk more about why the food you are eating today is not the same food your grandparents ate, but let this one statement sink in:

**THE VAST MAJORITY OF AMERICANS DO NOT GET THE AMOUNT OF POLY0PHENOLS OUR BODIES NEED TO PREVENT CHRONIC DISEASES.**

## TOP FOODS IN POLYPHENOL CONTENT IN MILLIGRAMS PER 100 GRAMS (FOUR OUNCES):

This French study shows how difficult it would be to get all the polyphenols you need from today's food.

| Food/ Seasoning | Polyphenols | Antioxidants |
|---|---|---|
| Cocoa Powder | 3,488 | 1,104 |
| Dark Chocolate | 1,664 | 1,860 |
| Flaxseed meal | 1,528 | Not Available |
| Black Elderberry | 1,359 | 1,950 |
| Chestnut | 1,215 | 2,757 |
| Blueberry | 836 | 471 |
| Black olive | 569 | 117 |
| Hazelnut | 495 | 687 |
| Pecan | 493 | 1,816 |
| Green olive | 346 | 411 |
| Strawberry | 235 | 268 |
| Red wine | 216 | Variable |

| Food/ Seasoning | Polyphenols | Antioxidants |
|---|---|---|
| Coffee | 214 | 267 |
| Black grape | 169 | 205 |
| Onion (red) | 168 | 91 |
| Apple | 136 | 205 |
| Spinach | 119 | 248 |
| Green tea | 89 | 62 |
| Black bean | 59 | 1,290 |

Let's step back a moment and take a look at what I consider to be the most important types of polyphenols and where you'll find them:

**Catechins:** Found in red wine, deep red colored fruits like grapes, raspberries, and cherries and their seeds as well as chocolate, apples, and broad beans. A subgroup of catechins called epigallocatechin is found in green tea in very large amounts (114 mg in four ounces). Dark chocolate (the kind without sugar!) is also a great source of catechins.

**Curcuminoids:** Curcuminoids (especially curcumin) are the medically active rhizome of the Indian spice turmeric, *Curcuma longa,* a plant in the ginger family, which has been used in traditional Indian medicine for millennia. Curcumin and turmeric give traditional Indian curries their characteristic bright yellow color. While you may find information that it is not easily absorbable by the human body, research shows that when it is processed in a very specific manner (BCM-95 formulation), curcuminoid polyphenols are very available for the body to use to combat inflammation

**Cyanidins:** Also found in deep red and purple fruits and vegetables, including black and red grapes, cherries, cranberries, elderberries, raspberries, and red onions. Cyanidins are also found in abundance in apples. The highest concentrations of cyanidins are found in the seeds. A subcategory of cyanidins, anthocyanidin and its subcategory proanthocyanidin, can give you a huge polyphenol boost. I'm especially a fan of oligomeric proanthocyanidins in French grape seed extract, probably the most powerful antioxidants known to science.

**Phenolic acids:** These powerful antioxidants are easily absorbed through the intestinal tract, making them especially effective in fighting against disease. They are found in abundance in yams, potato skins, garlic, Brussels sprouts, tomatoes, kale, and broccoli. Bee propolis, while not technically a food, is one of my favorite phenolic compounds, acts as a "glue" to seal beehives against infection and contamination. It does much the same thing in the human body. More to come.

## WHAT YOU NEED TO KNOW:

- Polyphenols are a grab bag of power nutrients that protect your body against the diseases of aging, including heart disease, cancer, diabetes, Alzheimer's disease, and many more.
- Several studies show that people who have the highest polyphenol intake live the longest.
- There are over 8,000 identified polyphenols occuring naturally in fruits and vegetables.
- The most colorful fruits and vegetables are often the best sources of polyphenols.

# CHAPTER 2
# Our Depleted Food Resources

Food is Mother Nature's way of caring for humans and all occupants of our planet, giving us exactly what we need to survive and thrive.

Sadly, human intervention has so severely disrupted the balance and the bounty that Mother Nature gives us. We must turn to other means of maintaining our health and retaining it if we have faltered.

Your Grandma's orange isn't the same as the one you eat today. Some experts estimate you would have to eat eight oranges today to get the same nutrition you would have gotten in an orange your grandma or great-grandma ate in 1950.

Case in point: The nutrient content of soils in the United States has severely declined in the past 70 years. Researchers who evaluated the content of essential vitamins and minerals in foods warned back in 2004 that modern farming methods have robbed soil—and food—of these critical nutrients. The study approved by the U.S. Department of Agriculture did not specifically evaluate polyphenol content since polyphenols are a Johnny-come-lately to the research world, but I think it's fair to assume that the decline in nutrients in foods translates equally when we're considering polyphenol content.

Among other things, the 2004 study found the riboflavin content of the 43 fruits and vegetables surveyed had declined by 38% between 1950 and 1999. (I know, these figures are old. That's because there doesn't seem to be much or even any scientific curiosity or urgency about the issue.)

So, let's take riboflavin as an example. Riboflavin, also known as vitamin B2, is key to the growth, development, and function of the 37.2 trillion cells in the human body. It's required for the proper development of skin, the lining of the digestive tract and blood and brain cells. Think of the damage such a dramatic loss of just one essential nutrient can do.

Agricultural researchers have raised the alarm about nutrient-depleted soils that can't grow optimally and produce foods that meet human nutritional needs. In 2017, Australian scientists found that due to intense, mismanaged farming, soil nutrients are declining all over the world. Nitrogen stores have decreased by 42 percent, phosphorus by 27 percent, and sulfur by 33 percent.

The 2004 study published in the *American Journal of Clinical Nutrition* included data from US Department of Agriculture databases found declines in levels of protein, calcium, phosphorus, iron, and vitamin C as well as riboflavin over the previous half century. I think it is fair to extrapolate those declines for other nutrients as well, including polyphenols. Now think of the hundreds of nutrients we get in our food, and you can see the serious impact soil depletion had on human health.

Why is this happening?

We can pretty much blame modern farming techniques driven by the quest for higher yields at any cost. That encouraged factory farming, deep plowing, excessive uses of fertilizers, pesticides and herbicides, all of which leach vital nutrients from the soil that would be passed on to crops in optimal conditions.

More enlightened farmers are now protecting soil from these losses and regenerating the nutrients lost by adding crop residues like straw, cornstalks, other stems and roots, and manure, and allowing time for fields to remain fallow so the soil can recover.

There is an encouraging trend toward no-till farming and replenishment of soils with winter crops and organic farming methods. It's even more encouraging that the US Department of Agriculture estimates that more than 35% of the eight major crops in the US are being farmed using the no-till method (not necessarily organically), thereby reducing the release of carbon stored in soil that contributes to greenhouse gases.

Let me add here that, of course, bee propolis is not a fruit or a vegetable, but its considerable polyphenol content makes it part of my recommended polyphenol cocktail. Bees carry wide varieties of pollen on their daily errands and healthy pollen makes healthy bees makes healthy propolis.

Still, this leads us to the obvious question: If the soils are so depleted, how can we get the nutrients our bodies need? Especially, how can we get the polyphenol intake so important to protect us from chronic diseases, aging in general, and from dying before our time?

That's where supplements become more and more essential to our wellbeing. In today's world, supplements are an important insurance policy for our health. This is true when they are made from top quality ingredients sustainably grown in rich soils that have been carefully nurtured to transfer the highest possible nutritional value to the fruits and vegetables they produce.

As I said in Chapter 1, I consider high quality supplements to be an insurance policy to guarantee my well-being in addition to my healthy diet and lifestyle.

# CHAPTER 3
# Curcumin: A Polyphenol Treasure Trove

What if I told you there is a polyphenol treasure trove that can give you the gift of a long and healthy life? How about an extract of this familiar spice that can prevent and even reverse heart disease, cancer, diabetes, Alzheimer's disease, depression, joint pain, and more?

Maybe you would think it's just a bunch of hype, but I can assure you there is voluminous scientific research that warrants placing curcumin at the pinnacle of all healing herbs.

If you love curry, you'll be familiar with turmeric, a popular, vividly colored spice. Inside turmeric is a compound called curcumin, which is found in its rhizome (the stem of the plant found underground). Curcumin is responsible for the golden orange color of turmeric and is perhaps the most powerful botanical medicine in the world today.

Botanically known as *Curcuma longa,* the turmeric rhizome is a member of the polyphenol-rich ginger family. You might be understandably skeptical when you hear that this humble Indian spice can prevent, treat, and cure a wide variety of serious diseases. These include everything from heart attacks to a dozen types of cancer, the pain of all types of arthritis and even so-called "incurable" diseases like diabetes and Alzheimer's. Curcumin also soothes depression and the agony of a variety of digestive disorders, including Crohn's disease, inflammatory bowel disease, and irritable bowel syndrome.

The unique polyphenolic flavonoids in curcumin are called curcuminoids, especially known for their anti-inflammatory, anticancer, and antitumor benefits. That pretty much checks all the boxes when it comes to chronic disease, which is why I am so enthusiastic about this humble rhizome.

## WHAT IS CURCUMIN AND HOW DOES IT WORK?

For centuries, curcumin has given the gift of long life and robust health to the people of India, for whom various types of curries—always made with turmeric and its important ingredient, curcumin—are a dietary staple. Curcumin is an important ingredient in the Ayurvedic medicine tradition and a vital part of Traditional Chinese Medicine (TCM). Now I can say without equivocation that it is the cure-all of the 21st century, backed by voluminous research that credits its healing powers to its exceptional antioxidant and anti-inflammatory effects.

Curcumin is one of the most powerful antioxidants known to science, hundreds of times more powerful than blueberries, which have substantial antioxidant capabilities themselves.

On the ORAC (Oxygen Radical Absorbance Capacity) scale that rates the antioxidant power of foods, only BCM-95® Curcumin rates over 1.5 million per 100 grams, while antioxidant- rich blueberries have only a 6,000 ORAC rating per 100 grams! This means that just one high-quality curcumin capsule delivers more than 25 times the antioxidants as the same amount of blueberries.

Curcumin literally scrubs the oxidative "rust" from your cells, preventing serious disease and reversing diseases you may already have. It helps stop cell deterioration and restores the cellular genetic codes to youthful levels, ensuring those cells will reproduce more like they did when you were young.

Inflammation is a factor in 80 to 90% of all disease, according to curcumin researcher Ajay Goel, Ph.D., director of Epigenetics and Cancer Prevention at Baylor University Medical Center in Dallas.

"Curcumin demonstrates superior antioxidant and anti-inflammatory effects and provides liver-and-heart-protective benefits as well. It is a potent antibacterial, antifungal, antiviral, anti-allergenic, and has antitumor and anti-cancer properties," says Dr. Goel.

By knocking out viruses, bacteria and fungi, curcumin offers the powerful possibility that we can use it to treat everything from colds and flu to pneumonia or even to help with something as serious as AIDS or cancer, effectively and without dangerous side effects.

In the case of cancer, cutting-edge research shows curcumin has a variety of ways of stopping abnormal cell growth, including an ability to affect cell division on the genetic level.

More important, from the viewpoint of damaged cell division found in cancer, curcumin also tells these cells to die when their time comes, as ordained by nature, which stops tumor growth.

In addition, curcumin has a unique ability to cross the blood-brain barrier, a membrane that protects the brain from invaders like bacterial infections and keeps out most other substances as well, including those that might be helpful. This gives curcumin the ability to deliver its antioxidants and anti-inflammatories directly to the brain, which is particularly helpful in cases of dementia and depression.

If that's not enough, studies also show that curcumin protects the liver and kidneys.

Curcumin has been compared to pharmaceutical drugs for the treatment of a wide variety of diseases and it has come out on top in every case.

What's not to love?

## ALL CURCUMIN IS NOT CREATED EQUAL

*However, there is very little curcumin in the spice turmeric.* If you've seen cheap turmeric and on the market, understand that they only contain 2 to 5% curcumin, which may or may not be usable by your body. They're not likely to have any effectiveness in terms of prevention or treatment for the diseases we're talking about.

Unless you are willing to eat curry three times a day for a lifetime, you probably can't eat enough turmeric or curcumin to make much of a difference to your health. Curcumin is *many times* more powerful than turmeric if you find the right formulation.

As my friend Dr. Goel says, "Turmeric is a spice, curcumin is a medicine."

In its most common form, even extracted curcumin is not very absorbable or bioavailable to the human body. It's especially difficult for the intestinal tract to retain the compounds long enough for them to be effective.

Fortunately, there is a highly absorbable and useful formulation called BCM-95 that brings curcumin's vast healing benefits into everyone's reach. The BCM-95 process combines with turmeric essential oil that has been well-researched and shown to be more than 700 times more absorbable and remains longer in the bloodstream than cheap formulations.

One of the things BCM-95 stands for is that a product contains 95% standardized levels of non-GMO turmeric curcuminoids grown and extracted without chemicals. In fact, BCM-95 is up to ten times more absorbable (and retained in the bloodstream longer at more medicinal levels) than standard 95% curcumin extracts. Only BCM-95 formulations have the turmeric essential oil coating and its main constituent, ar-turmerone to improve bioavailability and remain in the body for at least 8 hours. More than 70 scientific studies have confirmed the bioavailability of BCM-95 curcumin.

I recommend taking a product that provides 500 mg of pure curcuminoids per serving.

It's important to avoid curcumin supplements that contain piperine (black pepper). Once thought to boost the absorbability of curcumin, later research shows black pepper actually increases the possibility of some unpleasant side effects and interactions with commonly prescribed medications.

## WHAT YOU NEED TO KNOW:

- Curcumin and its potent polyphenol flavonoids, called curcuminoids, offers a health powerhouse.
- Scientific evidence confirms curcumin's antioxidant, anti-inflammatory, anticancer, antitumor benefits and much more.
- It has been proven effective in preventing and reversing at least ten types of cancer, heart disease, type 2 diabetes, depression, cognitive dysfunction, including Alzheimer's disease, degenerative arthritis, and more.
- The only truly effective supplements that are usable by the human body are those formulated using an extraction process called BCM-95.

# CHAPTER 4
# The Buzz on Propolis

Propolis is a bee product that has the unique honor of being an excellent source of polyphenols.

What's propolis? You may see it listed as an ingredient in your natural toothpaste or skin care products, cosmetics and cough syrups, and lozenges.

Propolis is the protector of the entire bee colony. Its name reflects its reason for being: pro—from the Latin "for" and polis, "the city." "For the city" is exactly what propolis does. Stay with me.

Can we take a moment here to navigate the complex world of a beehive?

A beehive is like a city with about 50,000 citizens, maintained year-round at a temperature of about 50 degrees Fahrenheit and 90% humidity. Honey is the hive's food. To keep the temperatures warm enough in winter, the bees cluster together and exercise their flight wings. They subsist on honey in the cold and scarce times. To accomplish this in cold climates, the colony must consume about two pounds of honey a week.

Propolis is a brown, sticky, waxy resin produced only by honeybees by mixing resins from leaf buds and tree sap flows with their saliva and beeswax. The bees load these sticky resins into the pollen baskets on their hind legs and carry them back to the hive. Sometimes called "bee glue," honeybees use propolis to repair and seal openings, damage, and cracks in their hives. Just like fixing the problem you might have with a drafty house in winter, bees would not survive winters without propolis.

It's also used to seal the cells in the honeycomb where the larvae grow to keep them safe and to ensure the future of the colony.

Propolis also has two other important functions:

It keeps the colony safe by forming barriers to keep out external enemies like snakes, mice, and lizards. In fact, if a predator manages to make its way into the hive, the worker bees immediately kill it and effectively mummify it with propolis so a body that is too heavy to remove is prevented from contaminating the hive as it decomposes.

And here's where we bring out the brass band—TA-DA! Propolis keeps the hive healthy by blocking all types of disease-and infection-causing microorganisms that would be expected to thrive in that 50-degree, high humidity environment.

Let me repeat that because it's so important:

***Propolis keeps the hive healthy by blocking all types of disease-and infection-causing microbes that would be expected to thrive in that 50-degree, high humidity environment.***

Researchers have identified more than 300 elements in propolis, most of them polyphenols.

The polyphenols in propolis come largely from the flavonoid category, produced as part of a plant's immune system and passed on by bees when they collect pollen and resin, and form propolis.

These potent compounds give propolis its ability to overcome invasion by viruses, bacteria and fungi.

And it's an excellent source of the anti-inflammatory polyphenolic compound called caffeic acid phenethyl ester.

Plus, propolis is a rich source of vitamins, minerals, enzymes, and essential oils.

Even though the leaf and tree sap sources for propolis may vary for honeybee colonies around the world, researchers find that colonies everywhere are protected by its impressive pathogen-fighting properties.

It's important to recognize that the conditions in a beehive—high humidity, and warm temperatures are quite similar to the human body's climate.

I'm talking about its nearly unparalleled antimicrobial properties. With the prevalence of rogue viruses in our world today, what could possibly be more important than a way to conquer viruses, bacteria, fungi, and other dangerous pathogens naturally and effectively?

Propolis is an incredibly complex molecule with hundreds of components. Its healing power comes mainly from phenolic compounds, like flavonoids (including quercetin, galangin, chrysin) and derivatives of another polyphenol group called hydroxycinnamic acids (caffeic acid, cinnamic acid, p-coumaric acid). Propolis also contains other healing molecules, including aromatic aldehydes, diterpenes, sesquiterpenes, esters, lignans, alcohols, amino acids, fatty acids, vitamins, and minerals.

Of course, in this time of rampant microbial attacks on humans, a natural substance that conquers viruses and harmful bacteria is a treasure. One that does all of this without the need for expensive laboratory tests and without side effects or a buildup of resistant microbes is a treasure beyond measure.

Beyond the natural antibiotic properties of propolis, propolis has long served humankind by helping heal wounds, even those that were severely infected.

It wipes out fungal and parasitic infections, making it a broad spectrum antimicrobial unparalleled in the world of natural healing. It's a powerful medicine against chronic allergics as well as providing the powerful anticancer properties found in polyphenols.

There is an abundance of other ailments against which propolis is a proven healer, including:

- *H. pylori* bacterial infections that cause gastric ulcers
- Burns
- Periodontal disease
- Tooth decay
- Vaginitis
- Acne
- *And more*

What's the common ground in the list above? They are all infections caused by harmful bacteria.

Viruses are the scourge of today's life no matter where on Earth you live. Since the pandemic changed all of our lives in March of 2020, it has presented challenges we never would have imagined. Many of us have contracted the coronavirus that causes Covid-19. Some have debilitating long-term effects. Sadly, too many of us have lost loved ones.

The peaks and valleys of contagion continue and are likely to have a profound impact on our lives for years, perhaps decades to come.

Propolis provides a promising answer to Covid-19 and the host of other viruses, including flu and colds, that plague humankind.

In fact, in just a short time, there has been credible published research on propolis as an effective method for treating and preventing Covid-19.

Propolis has long been recognized as a powerful, natural, antiviral treatment. Remember the bees and their use of propolis to keep all sorts of infections out of their hives and to clean them up, creating an almost sterile environment if pathogens were able to enter the hive? Well, propolis can do the same for the human organism as well.

Bees are vulnerable to a wide range of diseases, including at least 22 identified viruses.

Of course, humans are susceptible to many more viruses. We have all experienced the multitude of viruses that cause colds and flu at one time or another. Every single one of us has been affected by the SARS-CoV-2 viral infection that causes Covid.

But, how often do we think of other viral infections that have had such a profound impact?

How about HIV, the virus that causes AIDS? Or the HPV (human papillomavirus), a sexually transmitted disease that can result in several genital cancers? Or the viruses that cause hepatitis, Ebola, and dengue fever that periodically reach epidemic and even pandemic levels in scattered parts of the world?

Propolis has been studied and found to be safe and effective against all of them.

The Brazilian researchers who published a comprehensive review of published studies on the antiviral effects of propolis in early 2021 enthusiastically conclude that propolis works better than antiviral drugs that diminish their own effectiveness by triggering viral mutations and variations. Propolis has no known side effects, as opposed to antiviral drugs like acyclovir, interferon-a, and oseltamivir, that can cause kidney injury, neurological damage and more.

Propolis offers hope and, yes, even excitement.

Not only has propolis been proven effective against a wide range of bacterial infections, it doesn't create antibiotic resistance (because it isn't an antibiotic in the pharmaceutical sense). There are some cases in which propolis can enhance the effectiveness of pharmaceutical antibiotics against resistant bacteria.

Crucial 2018 study results confirmed that propolis is effective against the *Staphylococcus aureus* that causes potentially deadly MRSA, a highly contagious bacterial infection commonly found in hospitals and nursing homes. Better yet, repeated use of propolis in a lab setting did not result in any resistance.

Other US research confirmed the effectiveness of propolis against *Escherichia coli* and there is evidence it is effective against *Mycobacterium tuberculosis,* the bacteria that cause tuberculosis, a disease that is on the rise worldwide.

## PREVENT AND TREAT CANCER

Cancer is a complex disease that develops in many different ways and requires multiple types of treatment.

Propolis is a rich soup of anticancer nutrients, especially its flavonoid polyphenols including quercetin, chrysin, kaempferol, and apigenin. These have components that fight cancer in at least five ways (maybe more—new ones are being confirmed frequently!) and has been clinically proven to be effective at slowing, stopping or even eliminating cancer growth in some of the most-deadly forms of the disease.

This explains a part of the anticancer activity, since cellular oxidation is a major factor in almost all human diseases of aging, including cancer. Antioxidants, like the polyphenols in propolis, are well-studied and proven to prevent cancer and treat existing cancers as well as almost all other chronic diseases.

Propolis is well-studied and proven to be effective against the most common and the deadliest types of cancer. It works in a broad range of ways to prevent and treat cancer by:

- Boosting the immune system to fight off cancers before they begin
- Stopping wild cell division that forms tumors
- Telling those wild cells to die at the end of their normal lifespan
- Stopping the terrible disease-causing effects of free radical oxygen species
- Enhancing the effectiveness of conventional chemotherapy drugs.
- Stops the spread and re-emergence of cancer

## IN CONCLUSION...

Propolis is safe and effective for adults and children and is especially effective in combatting viruses like the flu, and yes, even the virus that causes Covid 19 as well as a vast range of bacterial, fungal, and other microbial infections.

If you are feeling ill, it's not necessary to define the cause of your illness because, unlike antibiotics or antivirals that only target specific infections, propolis can combat them all.

NOTE: There have been rare allergic reactions to propolis, mostly characterized by skin irritation that disappears as soon as you stop taking it.

## WHAT YOU NEED TO KNOW:

- Propolis is a sticky substance made by bees to protect hives from disease, infection and decaying materials that might invade the hive.

In humans, propolis has a wealth of polyphenols that:

- Protect against bacterial, fungal and viral infections
- Prevent and treating a variety of types of cancer
- Neutralize *H. pylori* bacterial infections that cause gastric ulcers
- Soothe and help heal burns
- Reverse periodontal disease
- Treat tooth decay and more

# CHAPTER 5
# The Magic of French Grape Seed Extract

Oligomeric proanthycyanidins – that's a tongue twister for sure. Let's call them OPCs for short. These unique polyphenols are the key to cancer prevention and reversal, heart health, cognitive health, and much more.

Although OPCs are polyphenols found in many plants, they are concentrated to extraordinary levels in grape seeds, hence their healing power.

My friend, Dr. Ajay Goel, a cancer researcher at City of Hope, is certainly impressed with this range of healthful benefits and especially with the cutting-edge research his team has completed that confirms its powerful activity against the deadliest cancers. In Dr. Goel's opinion and mine, French grape seeds are the best sources of these unique OPCs.

French grape seed comes from the royalty of grapes. Think of French wine and you'll quickly get the idea: There is nothing better!

Our ancestors loved wine fermented from grapes. Today's science has confirmed the health benefits of wine, many of which are derived from the seeds themselves. Concentrating those life-giving and even life-extending benefits into grape seed extract makes French grape seed extract (FGSE) a potent tool that should be part of every household's medicine cabinet, whether you are suffering from one of the many diseases of aging or if, like all of us, you want to avoid them altogether.

There are only a handful of botanicals known today that can achieve these remarkable healing feats:

- Reduce inflammation, an underlying factor in many chronic diseases
- Prevent and treat cancer by attacking it in several ways
- Lower blood pressure
- Strengthen and relax blood vessel walls
- Lower cholesterol and triglycerides
- Control blood sugars
- Help you lose weight
- Protect brain cells
- Protect memory by helping create neural pathways as alternative pathways to transmit information
- Strengthen the structure of bones and joints

Lab studies show that OPC polyphenols are much more effective in neutralizing destructive free radical oxygen molecules than vitamin C, vitamin E, and virtually any type of food.

The antioxidant levels in French grape seed extract are so high they are quite literally off the scale. The ORAC (oxygen racial absorbance capacity) value of FGSE is so high it is difficult even for modern equipment to accurately measure it. ORAC values are a measure of the free-radical fighting capabilities of a particular food.

We know that French grape seed extract has an ORAC value of at least 20,000 per gram, higher than any other food! Compare this to blueberries, which have a rating of 96 per gram, dark chocolate powder at 56 and strawberries at 43.

Foods with high antioxidant power, like French grape seed extract, balance immune system responses to reduce long-term (chronic) inflammation as well as short-term (acute) inflammation that governs wound healing and allergic responses. This has profound effects on virtually every chronic disease known to science.

Of course, we are talking about the *right* grape seed extract. In recent years, there have been some cheap products on the market that have little or no value. So-called grape seed extract from China can cost as little as $20 per kilo. In this case, you get what you pay for.

The best quality grape seed extract comes from tannin-free French OPC grapes that have a small molecular structure for the best absorbability—and the raw materials cost twenty times as much. It's truly worth it.

There's an extra bang for your buck in French grape seed extract.

## FIGHT CANCER

We know that some natural substances—like FGSE and the OPCs in it—can repair genetic damage and tell cancer-preventive genes to wake up and do their jobs. They signal genes that are overactive to calm down and behave in a normal manner rather than reproducing wildly. We know OPCs can also eliminate cancer stem cells, the main reason why even "successful" cancer treatment almost always ends with a recurrence.

Here's a synopsis of the wide number of ways that FGSE and its OPCs target cancer in a most impressive number of ways. It is scientifically proven to:

- Reduce tumor size
- Prevent cells from becoming cancerous
- Relieve inflammation, an underlying cause of cancer and many other chronic diseases
- Stop the formation of blood vessels that feed cancerous tumors (angiogenesis)
- Signal cancerous cells to commit suicide (apoptosis)
- Target cancer stem cells, the major reason why cancers spread (metastasis)
- Awaken sleeping genes that stop the growth of cancerous cells or slow down genes that are telling cells to reproduce wildly (epigenetics)
- Protect smokers

- Overcome the body's natural rejection of chemotherapy drugs over time (chemoresistance)
- Works synergistically with other natural treatments, including curcumin
- Enhance conventional chemotherapy treatments while protecting healthy cells and organs (chemoprotection)

FGSE's ability to fight cancer is applicable to the causes of other diseases, especially inflammation and epigenetics (genes that do not reproduce exactly due to environmental, not inherited factors).

## SYNERGY

I've mentioned synergy in earlier chapters—the combination of two or more ingredients that produce a result greater than the sum of the parts. The polyphenol powerhouse ingredients I present in this book all work synergistically, but probably none are so well-studied as the combination of the polyphenols found in FGSEs and curcumin.

Dr. Goel's research team found that if you add the OPCs in French grape seed extract to the verified anti-cancer powers of curcumin, we have a one-two punch against cancer that can't be beat.

In their study published in *Scientific Reports* in 2018, his team found that the botanical combination was doubly effective in preventing carcinogenesis (failures in cell reproduction that start the cancer process) and enhanced other anticancer weapons.

The results were so important that they concluded: "We make a case for the clinical co-administration of curcumin and OPCs as a treatment therapy for patients with colorectal cancer."

## LONG LIFE

Resveratrol is another antioxidant, another manifestation of the power of polyphenols, also found in grape skin (not the seed), berries and peanuts. It's known for its unique anti-aging, anti-inflammatory, and disease-fighting properties.

Substantial research shows that resveratrol has many of the same disease-fighting capabilities as OPCs. It just works in a slightly different way. There is also evidence that the two combined, as they are exclusively in French grape seed extract VX1, which was used in Dr. Goel's research, complement each other synergistically, enhancing their total power.

Studies show that resveratrol increases the lifespans of some animals (including yeast, worms, fruit flies, fish, and mice) who are fed a high-calorie diet, but resveratrol seems to trick their bodies into "thinking" that they are consuming a life-extending, low-calorie diet.

## THE RIGHT STUFF

French grape seed extract comes from grapes grown in the wine regions of France, where some of the world's finest wines are produced. They are rich sources of polyphenols, abundant plant nutrients that are the underlying source of protection against all of the diseases we've examined in this book.

The ideal French grape seed extract is free of tannins. While those tannins give wines their body and flavor, they are not absorbable, so they don't provide any health benefits. You don't want them in your grape seed extract.

The OPCs in other forms of grape seed extract typically are composed of a variety of weights and sizes. The large non-absorbable molecules in grape seed extract are known as condensed tannins, which have no health benefits and are not absorbed by the human body.

Cheaper forms of grape seed extract are often spiked with additional tannins intended to bulk them up, resulting in low prices and fewer health benefits since they cannot be used by the human body.

Look for a tannin-free product with a small molecular structure for maximum absorption.

Seek out a formulation called grape seed extract VX1, which has 99% polyphenols, 80% OPCs, and 27-32% dimers. If that sounds like a complicated search, let me reassure you that it's not complicated at all. A quick Google search will bring you to the right place.

## WHAT YOU NEED TO KNOW:

- Grape seed extract contains oligomeric proanthocyanidins (OPCs), potent polyphenols best known for their ability to combat cancer in a variety of ways.
- French grape seed extract is the most effective source of OPCs.
- In combination with curcumin. OPCs in French grape seed extract have a synergistic effect that is especially effective against several types of cancer.

There are only a handful of botanicals known today that can achieve these remarkable healing feats:

- Reduce inflammation, an underlying factor in many chronic diseases
- Prevent and treat cancer by attacking it in several ways
- Lower blood pressure
- Strengthen and relax blood vessel walls
- Lower cholesterol and triglycerides
- Control blood sugars
- Help you lose weight
- Protect brain cells
- Protect memory by helping create neural pathways as alternative pathways to transmit information
- Strengthen the structure of bones and joints

# CHAPTER 6
# An Apple a Day…

An apple a day keeps the doctor away. Our grandparents and great grandparents swore by the adage and it's still true today.

Apples are among the healthiest foods we can eat, and they can be even more healthy if we concentrate the flavonoid-rich peels into supplements.

Since we know that we're in a race to get all of the nutrients possible from our food that is so often grown in nutrient-depleted soil, apples as food and as supplements give us an easy answer.

Apples are high on the list of polyphenols that almost everyone enjoys and eats regularly. They're inexpensive and easily available almost anywhere in the world, so it's not a stretch to consciously add them to your healthy diet.

Several studies confirm that apple consumption is directly related to longer life expectancy, perhaps as much as 12% longer. That means an extra 9.24 years of life for the average American, who can now expect to live 77 years.

Those apple flavonoids, polyphenols to the max, are great sources of disease-preventing antioxidants and the anti-inflammatory benefits that go with them. Apples are particularly rich in the subclasses of flavonoids, including flavonols, flavones, and flavanols.

Apples are also rich sources of oligomeric proanthycyanidins (OPCs) like those found in red grapes. They are also rich sources of the polyphenols, quercetin, catechins, phloridzin, and chlorogenic acid, all of which are strong antioxidants.

While we all love to bite into a ripe juicy apple, like in many fruits and vegetables, the highest flavonoid content is in the skin. Similar to the benchmark in many fruits and vegetables, the dark and more vibrant the color, the more polyphenols are present in an apple. There is some variability in the polyphenol potency in different varieties of apples, but if you gravitate toward dark red ones rather than green or yellow ones, you'll get the biggest benefits.

## HEART HEALTHY

Apple flavonoids are especially noted for their ability to block fat and cholesterol from entering the body and clogging arteries, an attribute of their polyphenol content as well as the pectin, a non-soluble fiber noted for its heart-healthy benefits.

In a study published in 2007, Japanese researchers confirmed that overweight people who took a supplement made from apple peels for just 12 weeks "significantly" reduced their cholesterol levels.

In addition to promoting healthy cholesterol levels

and preventing artery clogging fatty deposits, Spanish researchers very recently confirmed what Grandma knew: An apple a day can lower your blood pressure, make arteries more flexible, and control inflammation-causing cytokines that can lead to heart attacks, heart failure, and even sudden cardiac death.

## CANCER PREVENTION

Several studies confirm that women who eat apples regularly have a lower risk of developing several types of cancer, primarily lung cancer.

The Nurse's Health Study, that began three generations back in 1976 with more than 120,000 participants, set in stone the concept that fruit and vegetable consumption are directly connected to long, healthy lives, especially for women.

In 2016, Italian researchers found that apple consumption is specifically connected to protection against several types of cancer in *both* men and women. This includes up to 41% reduction in various gastrointestinal cancers (like stomach, colorectal, and esophageal cancers) and breast cancer.

Apple polyphenols protect against cancer by stopping or slowing the formation of cancerous cells and tumors—stopping the wild production of cancerous cells—usually the case in cancer. This protection stops the formation of blood vessel networks that feed the cancerous cells, stops metastasis or the spread of cancerous cells to other parts of the body, and improves general immune system function.

## BLOOD SUGAR CONTROL

Apple skins also contain a polyphenol called phloridzin, which is especially active against glycation or impaired glucose metabolism, one of the most common, preventable, and reversible causes of aging.

Phloridzin slows the process of glycation and its destructive effects, called advanced glycation end products (AGEs) at many different levels. For example, almost as soon as you consume a carbohydrate-containing meal that could cause a dangerous post-meal spike in blood sugar, phloridzin goes to work by coating lining of the small intestine and preventing the glucose from entering your bloodstream. Studies show that phloridzin inhibits glucose uptake by 52%.

## WEIGHT CONTROL

Apples are low in caloric density, meaning they contain lots of water and relatively few calories. They are loaded with fiber, so they are filling and satisfyingly sweet. This makes them an excellent weight control tool, although they may specifically cause you to lose only a pound a year or so. What the fiber and pectin in apples can do is to help you feel full, so you don't splurge on high-calorie foods.

Duke Medical School's newsletter reported in 2011 that an apple a day can help prevent the accumulation of visceral fat, abdominal fat that can surround deep organs (even if you have a flat belly) and contributes to all of the chronic diseases we all want to avoid.

Quercetin, one of the powerhouse polyphenols, also plays a role in weight control, at least with apples, since its anti-inflammatory properties can reduce insulin resistance, which is closely linked to obesity. With insulin resistance, our bodies keep producing more insulin to counteract the glucose we take in and that excess insulin circulating through our bodies makes us fat. That is at least part of the reason why so many people with Type 2 diabetes are overweight.

## THERE'S MORE

Apple polyphenols offer effective tools for improving physical endurance and reducing fatigue.

They can help reduce allergy symptoms, including skin irritation and rashes, inflamed sinuses, and runny noses.

In combination with other botanicals, including French grape seed extract, they have been shown to improve men's libido and sexual performance.

Apple extracts are just as effective at offering you these benefits as the ones that came from the tree in Grandma's back yard.

## WHAT YOU NEED TO KNOW:

Apples are a key nutrient in human health offering a wealth of polyphenols that can:

- Promote longer lifespans in general
- Lower cholesterol
- Help control high blood pressure
- Prevent specific types of cancer
- Help control blood sugars
- Promote weight control
- Improve physical endurance
- Reduce fatigue
- Address allergy symptoms
- Improve men's libido and sexual performance

# CHAPTER 7
# Healthy Long Life with Green Tea

After water, tea is the most popular beverage in the world. It's also the key to health and long life because of its wealth of polyphenols.

When we talk about tea, I'm specifically referring to the leaves of the *Camellia sinensis* plant. It's a little-known secret that green tea and black tea come from the same shrub. They are simply processed differently.

And they both contain a treasure trove of polyphenols, but when it comes to the greatest contributions to your health, green tea wins hands down.

The *Camelia sinensis* plant is actually a shrub, grown largely in China and other parts of southeast Asia and India. It is a rich source of flavonols, flavanols, flavandiols, flavonoids, and phenolic acid. The most abundant polyphenols are a particular type of flavonols known as catechins, and the subcategory known as epigallocatechin-3-gallate (it's more simply known as EGCG).

EGCG is a powerful antioxidant, well researched for its broad capabilities to boost metabolism, encourage heart health, and stop a wide variety of types of cancer.

Green tea is steamed immediately after the green leaves are harvested, preventing them from fermenting and preserving the polyphenols, especially EGCG. Green tea is light green in color and has a mild flavor but has a plethora of polyphenol benefits not available in the stronger tasting black tea.

The leaves used to make black tea are rolled and allowed to oxidize and ferment. This process enhances the flavor and darkens the color, but also destroys some of the most important polyphenols that make green tea the healthier addition to your diet and your supplement plan. Black tea does contain some polyphenols and especially theaflavins, known for heart protective and blood sugar lowering properties, but their benefits pale in comparison to green tea.

I'm reaching for a big mug of green tea as I write this. I've already added a supplement containing green tea to my daily regimen.

Here are a few of the most exciting ways green tea works to preserve health, help you regain health and live a long and healthy life.

## DIABETES, BLOOD SUGAR, AND WEIGHT CONTROL

You are probably already aware that about 95% of people with type 2 diabetes are overweight. Extra pounds and especially dangerous belly fat can make blood sugar control worse in people with what was once known as adult-onset diabetes. Now, many children and teenagers are afflicted with the disease, primarily because of the epidemic of obesity among our young people.

Pivotal Chinese human research published in 2014 confirmed that green tea consumption, in either liquid or supplement form, had a significant effect on reducing insulin resistance and improving blood glucose levels in people diagnosed with Type 2 diabetes.

Whether or not you have diabetes or pre-diabetes, if you've got a few extra pounds (most of us do!), green tea can help you on the way to a healthy weight. It is a rich source of metabolism boosting EGCG that helps reduce belly fat and can give you a small, but significant boost in weight loss. Better yet, EGCGs have been shown to help maintain a healthy body weight once you've shed those extra pounds.

Part of the EGCG weight control formula is green tea's natural level of caffeine, another polyphenol known to help boost metabolism.

## HEART DISEASE

Heart disease is the leading cause of death in both men and women worldwide. Green tea has been well-researched as a way to combat heart disease by combatting the formulation of artery-clogging plaque, controls blood fats, and cholesterol.

British researchers found that EGCG helps dissolves those amyloid plaques, which are made of much the same substance as the plaques typical of Alzheimer's disease, reducing them to smaller soluble molecules that are less like to damage blood vessels and cause heart attacks and strokes.

Green tea has also been shown to reduce blood pressure, another factor in heart attacks and strokes.

## ALZHEIMER'S DISEASE

In addition to the abilities of EGCG to unclog blocked arteries, the same British research confirms that the amyloid plaques found in the brains of people with Alzheimer's disease can also be dissolved by drinking green tea or taking green tea supplements that concentrate the quantities of EGCG.

A Japanese review of current research on green tea and cognitive impairment, including Alzheimer's, confirms the theory that EGCG can prevent the development of dementia and slow the progress of the disease.

## CANCER

Green tea has been well studied in animal, lab and human studies for its effectiveness against several types of cancer, including breast, skin, lung, esophageal, colon, and bladder cancers.

According to the National Cancer Institute, EGCG and its close cousin, epigallocatechin, ECG, another catechin found in green tea, are strong antioxidants that protect cells from free radical damage. It protects cells against DNA damage that can generate cancer cells as well as stopping the formation of cancer tumors, encouraging the natural death of cells that wildly reproduce called apoptosis and starving cancer cells of the blood supply they need to grow and reproduce, a process called angiogenesis.

## A LITTLE BIT MORE, OR A LOT MORE...

If that's not enough to convince you that green tea should be a regular part of your healthy lifestyle, consider this:

- Green tea has been known to protect the liver by protecting against deadly fatty liver disease caused by a high fat diet.
- Its antibacterial properties are due to its ability to destroy cell walls of harmful bacteria and possibly slow or halt the transmission of viruses.
- It can increase your stamina. Animal studies showed that mice given green tea could swim four times as long as those who were green tee-totallers.
- It seems contradictory, but green tea, despite its caffeine content, has a calming effect by

interacting with brain receptors that help you chill out.
- Green tea blocks UV radiation and reduces sun damage on your skin, potentially preventing skin cancer as well as increasing collagen production of healthy skin and joints.
- It fosters better communication between the hemispheres of the brain.

## IF THAT'S NOT ENOUGH...

Japanese researchers studied more than 40,000 people with Type 2 diabetes and found that those who drank five or more cups of green tea a day were 15% less likely to die from any cause than those who drank a cup or less a day.

Better yet, another Japanese study that followed more than 46,000 people for more than 18 years found that green tea drinkers (up to six cups a day) were an astounding 27% less likely to die of any cause, even those who had already had a heart attack or a stroke!

## HOW TO GET THAT LIFE SURGE

If you're going to drink tea, I recommend about three cups a day, brewed for only about three minutes. The catechins lose their effectiveness the longer the tea sits, which is why those bottled and canned green tea drinks are basically useless.

Look for an organic variety without preservatives.

Green tea is an acquired taste, I can tell you. If it's not for you or you just want to increase your protection from this stellar polyphenol, I recommend a supplement.

## WHAT YOU NEED TO KNOW:

Green tea contains a powerhouse of polyphenols called catechins that can:

- Help with weight and blood sugar control and help control Type 2 diabetes
- Lower blood pressure and cholesterol
- Dissolve the dangerous plaque that blocks arteries and causes Alzheimer's disease
- Prevent and help control several types of cancer in several ways
- Protect your liver
- Stop bacterial infections and possibly control the spread of viruses
- Protect skin against UV damage
- Help generate collagen in skin and joints
- Promote a long healthy life by reducing death rates from all causes

# CHAPTER 8
# Other Fun Sources of Polyphenols

In Chapter 1, I introduced you to some of the polyphenols I consider most important, but here's the rub: There are more than 8,000 polyphenols. That doesn't mean you need to eat 8,000 foods in order to get all those important nutrients. Not at all!

All fruits and vegetables are great sources of polyphenols, but some are superstars. Cloves, cocoa, dark chocolate, black olives, and coffee are polyphenol powerhouses. That means they contain a multitude of nutrients that can act synergistically to enhance your health.

If you're not familiar with the term "synergistic," it means that the combination of two things equals more than simply adding the benefits together. It's sort of like 2+2=8. New math!

Remember in Chapter 1, I outlined a handful of the most important polyphenols?

You already know that fruits and vegetables are an essential part of your diet for a wide variety of reasons. They're antioxidants, preventing the degenerative diseases of aging like Type 2 diabetes, heart disease, cancer, Alzheimer's, and more.

But there's a magical synergistic combination here that prevents disease and premature death.

Let's take a deeper look at some unexpectedly healthy foods that display this type of synergy and give you a huge health bang for your buck. No, you don't have to eat handfuls of cloves, although they are nature's richest source of polyphenols per 300 grams—about four ounces—but who eats that many cloves?

Let's get real!

How about starting some faves for almost everyone? Who doesn't love chocolate, coffee, and red wine? I'm sure you're applauding these healthy choices. You may be surprised at the health benefits of some of these foods outside the norms of fruits and vegetables, which I know you're eating in big quantities every day, right?

## COFFEE

We've already established that caffeine is a polyphenol. Coffee is a great source of caffeine—a polyphenol that has exceptionally strong antioxidant and disease-preventing effects, with limits, of course.

In addition to caffeine, coffee is a rich source of chlorogenic acid, diterpenes, and trigonelline. Those terms probably don't mean much to you, but their antioxidant, anti-inflammatory, anticancer, anti-diabetes, and anti-hypertensive benefits are health-promoting winners.

One of the greatest gifts of chlorogenic acid is its clinically proven ability to combat metabolic syndrome, a demon's basket of insulin resistance, elevated blood pressure and cholesterol, and excess abdominal fat—all things that make you a sitting duck for diseases we want to avoid at all costs. And that's just one aspect of coffee.

Here are some others:

***Diterpenes***: The compounds are the basis for biologically important compounds such as retinol, retinal, and phytol. They are anti-inflammatory, protecting against the inflammation that is the underlying cause of so many chronic diseases, and antimicrobial, helpful against viral, bacterial, and fungal infections.

***Trigonelline***: This powerhouse helps keep blood sugars under control, manages cholesterol and blood fats, helps keep you calm and better able to manage stress, prevents migraines, fights bacterial and viral infections, stops tumor formation, eases migraines, and puts the brakes on the hearing loss often associated with type 2 diabetes. It prevents blood clotting that can cause heart attacks and strokes. Best of all, trigonelline has been linked with improving memory, a concern for all of us as we age.

By the way, you remember that I recommended eating the rainbow and brightly colored foods to get the highest levels of polyphenols? Well, the coffee beans you buy here in the US are brown because they have been dried and roasted. When the fruit is picked, it is a brilliant color of yellow, orange or red, depending on the variety.

So, feel free to stock up on a couple of cups of coffee a day. More isn't necessary or necessarily beneficial.

If you're not a huge fan of coffee (really?) try these other delicious beverages that offer similar benefits: green and black tea (they're actually from the same plant, just processed differently) and beer. I told you that you'd be surprised.

## CHOCOLATE

We're talking about the cacao plant here, grown mostly in Central and South America and Africa.

I have a friend who refers to her nightly "indulgence" in a square of rich dark chocolate as "taking my heart pill." That's not at all off base since the polyphenols in chocolate make it one of the most heart healthy foods you can find.

***Catechins:*** Largely applauded for their anti-inflammatory benefits, catechins are also a crucial element of weight control. Just remember that we're talking about *dark* chocolate here—that means low in sugar. Pure chocolate with sugar is extremely bitter, but you can easily find an 87% dark chocolate bar that will give you the catechin benefit without much sugar. Sugar is a no-no for a wide variety of reasons. Yes, that prohibition includes milk chocolate. You'll also find catechins in abundance in red wine, red grapes, and other deep red-colored foods. By the way, in their raw state, cacao beans are dark red.

Green tea is also a great source of catechins because of its signature epigallocatechin-3 gallate (ECGC). Stay with me, I'll get into that more in a page or two.

***Flavonol glycosides:*** Well-respected for their antioxidant activity, especially against diabetes and cancerous tumor growth, flavonol glycosides offer serious protective benefits in the form of a real treat.

***Anthocyanins and proanthocyanidins***: Maybe there's a good reason why we give chocolate on Valentine's Day, since these two power-packed polyphenols are great for heart health. They help boost the levels of nitric acid in the bloodstream relaxing blood vessels and lowering blood pressure. Not only are they excellent antioxidants, but they also block the formation of cancer-causing nitrosamines found in processed meats. Combined with vitamin C— (think dark chocolate with an orange—yum!)—these polyphenols have been shown to reduce the risk of breast cancer.

Chinese researchers found that those who eat dark chocolate had an overall lower risk of death from any cause. Eat up, in moderation, of course!

## RED WINE

Red wine is a repository of most of the benefits I've outlined in coffee and chocolate and then some. Made from deep red grapes, it is, of course, a rich source of catechins and proanthocyanidins, making them exceptionally valuable in combatting heart disease and cancer.

There's something called the French paradox. It goes something like this: The death rate from heart disease in France is very low considering their diet high in saturated fats and the high incidence of smoking. It's actually only about 25% of the death rates in Britain. The explanation? It's long been the theory that the red wine they typically consume with lunch and dinner has a protective effect.

That was confirmed in an iconic 2009 study from Yale that concluded that physicians could confidently recommend a glass or two of red wine daily for their patients. In addition to this recommendation, they confirmed that one or two drinks of red wine a day were significantly protective against death from all causes, especially for men, and against death from heart disease in both men and women.

Why not white wine? The polyphenol content of white wine is only about 10% of that found in red wine, the Yale scientists found.

Red wine is a trifecta of polyphenols: phenolic acids, flavonoids and stilbenes, especially the much-revered "longevity nutrient" resveratrol. These power nutrients are protective against virtually all the chronic disease associated with the Western diet high in saturated fats and processed foods.

There's something as yet undetermined in the fermentation process that seems to enhance the polyphenol content of red wine. But if you're not a wine drinker, not to worry. Resveratrol is found in peanuts, cocoa and, of course, red grapes, and grape seeds.

As with coffee and chocolate and even more so with wine, there's a fine line here, my friends. A little bit can be good, very good. Too much can increase health risks rather dramatically. In the case of red wine, moderate consumption is one five-ounce glass of red wine daily and two glasses for men under 65. Just one more drink a day increases the risk and more than five glasses a day becomes a high risk of heart disease and death.

In conclusion, you'll find polyphenols virtually everywhere in the plant world and in some places where you might not expect them. A diet rich in fresh fruits and vegetables is the healthiest possible, so enjoy yourself! And, as you'll see in the next chapter, give serious consideration to supplementing that healthy diet since we know that the polyphenol and other nutrient content of many foods is less than optimal.

## WHAT YOU NEED TO KNOW:

Polyphenols are found in all plant materials, and in some more than others.

- You might be surprised to find that coffee, chocolate, and red wine are all exceptionally high in polyphenol content.
- Polyphenols are universally antioxidant and anti-inflammatory.
- Polyphenols found in coffee have a unique effectiveness in preventing and fighting diabetes, cancer, and heart disease.
- Polyphenols in chocolate are especially effective anti-inflammatories, addressing the underlying causes of most chronic diseases.
- The polyphenols in red wine have been study-proven to increase lifespan and they're especially protective against heart disease and death from cardiovascular events like heart attacks and strokes.
- Consider supplements to ensure that you get the full value of polyphenols.

# CHAPTER 9
# Putting it All Together

So, we have here a combination of the most powerful polyphenols that will absolutely make a difference in your day-to-day quality of life, your overall health and your longevity. I can say that without equivocation because I've used these ingredients for years.

## SYNERGY

Synergy is the operative concept here.

Wikipedia defines synergy as "an interaction or cooperation giving rise to a whole that is greater than the simple sum of its parts."

The concept has its roots in the Greek word "syn-ergos," meaning "working together.

I couldn't describe the effects of the five main ingredients in my polyphenol cocktail any better: They work together to produce a result that is far greater than the individual health benefits of the already awesomely effective individual components.

**The five main ingredients in my polyphenol cocktail work together to produce a result that is far greater than the individual health benefits of the already awesomely effective individual components.**

## THE RECIPE

Here's a quick recap of the five main ingredients of the powerhouse polyphenol combo and what you should look for in order to find that magical synergy. All of them are powerful anti-inflammatories and antioxidants that trigger healing and prevention of chronic diseases in ways that science is uncovering nearly every day. Of course, our ancestors knew the medicinal properties of these common botanicals centuries ago. It's interesting, and perhaps comforting, that science is finally catching up with ancient wisdom.

### *CURCUMIN*

You'll remember that curcumin is the rhizome (underground stem) of the *Curcuma longa,* the turmeric plant, a member of the polyphenol-rich ginger family. It's an incredibly potent medicinal with a wide range of benefits, including its ability to fight cancer in a variety of ways not known in any other substance, botanical or pharmaceutical.

Curcumin's unique polyphenols called curcuminoids have been proven to prevent, treat and cure a wide variety of serious diseases, including everything from heart attacks to a dozen types of cancer, the pain of all types of arthritis and even so-called "incurable" diseases like diabetes and Alzheimer's. Curcumin also soothes depression and the agony of a variety of digestive disorders, including Crohn's disease, inflammatory bowel disease, and irritable bowel syndrome.

There are dozens, perhaps hundreds of curcumin products on the market today. Many of them are worthless because they cannot be used by the human body (they are not bioavailable).

Some products unexplainably contain piperine, essentially black pepper, an ingredient that was found to increase bioavailability in just one widely discredited study decades ago.

The only curcumin that has been scientifically proven to be bioavailable and effective in prevention and treatment of these disease is the BCM-95™ formulation. The BCM-95 process combines with turmeric essential oil that has been well-researched and shown to be more than 700 times more absorbable and remains longer in the bloodstream than cheap formulations. Only BCM-95 formulations have the turmeric essential oil coating and its main constituent, ar-turmerone to improve bioavailability and remain in the body for at least 8 hours. More than 70 scientific studies have confirmed the bioavailability of BCM-95 curcumin.

Please don't waste your money on anything else.

### *PROPOLIS*

This bee product protects the hive from infection and decay, and it will do the same for you.

Propolis is a brown, sticky, waxy resin produced only by honeybees by mixing resins from leaf buds and tree sap flows with their saliva and beeswax.

Sometimes called "bee glue," honeybees use propolis to repair and seal openings, damage, and cracks in their hives. Propolis keeps the hive healthy by blocking all types of disease-and infection-causing microorganisms that would be expected to thrive in the hive's 50-degree, high humidity environment.

Propolis is a high-quality source of anti-inflammatory polyphenolic compound called caffeic acid phenethyl ester.

Propolis is an incredibly complex molecule with hundreds of components with nearly unparalleled antimicrobial properties and has been found to be profoundly effective in treating a broad range of bacterial and viral infections.

### *FRENCH GRAPE SEED EXTRACT*

You'll remember that much of the potent healing power of French grape seed extract lies in the extraordinarily strong oligomeric proanthycyanidins, polyphenols that are the key to cancer prevention and reversal, heart health, cognitive health, and much more.

French grape seed extract has been scientifically validated to balance immune system responses to reduce long-term (chronic) inflammation as well as short-term (acute) inflammation that governs wound healing and allergic responses. This has profound effects on virtually every chronic disease known to science.

Of course, we are talking about the *right* grape seed extract. In recent years, there have been some cheap products on the market that have little or no value. So-called grape seed extract from China can cost as little as $20 per kilo. In this case, you get what you pay for.

The best quality grape seed extract comes from tannin-free, French OPC grapes that have a small molecular structure for the best absorbability—and the raw materials cost twenty times as much. It's truly worth it.

### *APPLE*

Apples have long been considered among the healthiest foods we can eat. Just ask your grandma who lived by the adage: An apple a day keeps the doctor away.

Apples are rich sources of oligomeric proanthycyanidins (OPCs) like those found in red grapes. They are also rich sources of the polyphenols quercetin, catechins, phloridzin and chlorogenic acid, all of which are strong antioxidants.

Extensive research confirms that apple polyphenols protect against heart disease and cancer, lowers blood sugar levels helping prevent and control Type 2 diabetes, helps control allergies, improve physical endurance for men's sexual health and are a great tool for weight control.

I believe Grandma was right: An apple a day is the key to a long and healthy life.

Apple extracts are a concentrated form of the red juicy ones we like to munch on and they are a great insurance policy against nutrients grown in depleted soil that may or may not be sufficient to give you the polyphenol protection you need.

### *GREEN TEA*

Green tea from the *Camellia sinensis* plant is a rich source of flavonols, flavanols, flavandiols, flavonoids, and phenolic acid, especially epigallocatechin-3-gallate, more simply known as EGCG. This powerful antioxidant is well researched for its broad capabilities to boost metabolism, encourage heart health and stop a wide variety of types of cancer.

Green tea is particularly revered for its ability to boost metabolism, an important factor when it comes to fighting obesity, controlling blood sugar and addressing the underlying causes of Type 2 diabetes.

Well-designed research confirms that EGCG can dissolve the amyloid plaques found in the brains of people with Alzheimer's disease.

Green tea extract is a good way of being sure you are getting that all-important EGCG and other polyphenols.

## ALL TOGETHER

I think you can easily see the value of these powerhouse nutrients. Physical vigor and stamina, mental focus and well-being, robust immune response, cardiovascular strength, and protection against cancer are just a few of the way's polyphenols are our best sources for vibrant health.

Individually, each of these ingredients is amazingly effective. Together, they are your best insurance policy against chronic disease and an assurance of a long and healthy life.

If for some reason you are unable to eat 5 or more servings of fruits and vegetables daily, I would highly recommend taking a supplement that may provide you with a high concentration of polyphenols similar to eating plenty of fruits and vegetables. Here is a formula that I love to take when I just can't get enough fruits and vegetables daily, curcumin, apple extract, green tea, propolis, and grape seed extract. I take this formula every day, it gives you plenty of polyphenols just like an abundance of eating fruits and vegetables.

Look for a synergistic blend of these five stellar sources of polyphenols that contains at least 250 mg of high-quality polyphenols per serving.

# References

**Chapter 1: Eat the Rainbow**

Zamora-Ros, Rabassa M, Cherubini A et al. High concentrations of a urinary biomarker of polyphenol intake are associated with decreased mortality in older adults. J Nutr. 2013 Sep;143(9):1445-50.

Russo G-L, Panuolo C, Russo M et al. Mechanisms of aging and potential role of selected polyphenols in extending healthspan. *Biochem Pharmacol.* 2020 Mar;173:113719.

**Chapter 2: Our Depleted Food Resources**

Davis DR, Epp MD. Changes in USDA food composition data for 43 garden crops, 1950 to 1999. *J Am Coll Nutr.* 2004 Dec;23(6):669-82.

Kopittke PM, Dalal RC, Finn D et al. Global changes in soil stocks of carbon, nitrogen, phosphorus, and sulphur as influenced by long-term agricultural production. *Glob Chang Biol.* 2017 Jun;23(6):2509-2519

**Chapter 3: Curcumin: A Polyphenol Treasure Trove**
Toden, S, Goel A. The Holy Grail of Curcumin and its Efficacy in Various Diseases: Is Bioavailability Truly a Big Concern? *Journal of Restorative Medicine* 2017; 6:27.

Oney-Montalvo J, Uc-Varguez A et al. Influence of Soil Composition on the Profile and Content of Polyphenols in Habanero Peppers (Capsicum chinense Jacq.) *Agronomy* 2020, 10(9), 1234.

**Chapter 4: The Buzz on Propolis**
Paspuleti VR, Sammugam L, Ramesh N et al. Honey, Propolis, and Royal Jelly: A Comprehensive Review of Their Biological Actions and Health Benefits. *Oxid Med Cell Longev* 2017; 2016: 1259510.

Ripari N, Sartori AA, Honorio MS et al. Propolis antiviral and immunomodulatory activity: a review and perspectives for Covid-19 treatment. *J Pharm Pharmacol.* 2021 Feb 8 : rgaa067.

Syamsudin PS, Djamil R, Heffen W et al. Apoptosis of human Breast Cancer Cells induced by Ethylacetate Extracts of Propolis. *American Journal of Biochemistry and Biotechnology* 6 (2): 84–88.

**Chapter 5: The Magic of French Grape Seed Extract**
Toden S, Ravindranathan P, Gu J et al. Oligomeric proanthocyanidins (OPCs) target cancer stem-like cells

and suppress tumor organoid formation in colorectal cancer. *Sci Rep*. 2018 Feb 20;8(1):3335.
Ravindranathan P, Pasham D, Balaji U et al. A combination of curcumin and oligomeric proanthycyanidins offer superior anti-tumorigenic properties in colorectal cancer. *Scientific Reports* 2018 Sep 14;8(1):13869.

**Chapter 6: An Apple a Day...**

Fabiani R, Minelli L et al. Apple intake and cancer risk: a systematic review and meta-analysis of observational studies. *Public Health Nutr* . 2016 Oct;19(14):2603-17.

Yuan C, Ng K. Can an apple a day keep cancer away? *Am J Clin Nutr.* 2021 Jun 1;113(6):1388-1389.

**Chapter 7: A Healthy Long Life With Green Tea**

Shirakami Y, Shimiizu M. Possible Mechanisms of green tea and. Its constituents against cancer. *Molecules*. 2018 Sep 7;23(9):2284.

Cooper R, Morre DJ et al. Medicinal benefits of green tea: part II. review of anticancer properties. *J Altern Complement Med.* 2005 Aug;11(4):639-52.

Renfan X, Yang K et al. Effect of green tea supplementation blood pressure: a systematic review and metanalysis of randomized controlled trials. *Medicine* (Baltimore) 2020 Feb; 99(6): e19047.

Liu CY, Huang CJ et al. Effects of Green Tea Extract on Insulin Resistance and Glucagon-Like Peptide 1 in Patients with Type 2 Diabetes and Lipid Abnormalities: A Randomized, Double-Blinded, and Placebo-Controlled Trial.PLoS One 2014; 9(3): e91163.

**Chapter 8: Other Fun Sources of Polyphenols**

Yamagata K. Do Coffee Polyphenols Have a Preventive Action on Metabolic Syndrome Associated Endothelial Dysfunctions? An Assessment of the Current Evidence. *Antioxidants* (Basel) 2018. Feb; 7(2): 26.

Fukushima Y, Tashiro T et al. Coffee and beverages are the major contributors to polyphenol consumption from food and beverages in Japanese middle-aged women. *J Nutr Sci*. 2014; 3: e48.

Zhong GC, Hu TY et al. Chocolate consumption and all-cause and cause-specific mortality in a US population: a post hoc analysis of the PLCO cancer screening trial. *Aging* 2021;13:14:18564-18585.

Cordova AC, Sumpio BE. Polyphenols are medicine: Is it time to prescribe red wine for our patients? *Int J Angiol*. 2009 Autumn; 18(3): 111–117.

# About the Author

## TERRY LEMEROND

Terry Lemerond is a natural health expert with over 50 years of experience helping people live healthier, happier lives. A much sought-after speaker and accomplished author, Terry shares his wealth of experience and knowledge in health and nutrition through his educational programs, including the Terry Talks Nutrition website TerryTalksNutrition.com—newsletters, pod- casts, webinars, and personal speaking engagements. Terry has also hosted Terry Talks Nutrition radio for the past 30 years. His books include:

*Fight Disease With A Powerful Natural Seed–The Wonders of French Grape Seed Extract*

*Andrographis–The Natural Answer to Disease*

*Type 2 Diabetes? Break Free Naturally, with Hintonia*

*Wake UP! Melatonin is For More Than Just Sleep*

*Relieve Pain without Side Effects*

*Trauma Comfrey, Nature's Healing Herb*

*Drug-Free Relief of Anxiety & Stress*

*Propolis, The Natural Way to Prevent and Heal Infection: Fights Infection Including: Bacterial, Viral, Fungal, Parasitic, and More*

*Seven Keys to Vibrant Health*

*Seven Keys to Unlimited Personal Achievement*

*50+ Natural Health Secrets Proven to Change Your Life*

Terry continues to author and co-author books to educate everyone on the steps they can take to live a healthier, vibrant life.

His continual dedication, energy, and zeal are part of his ongoing mission—to help us all improve our health.

# More about TTN Publishing, LLC

Everyone has the same desire:
a vibrant, healthy life!

TTN Publishing exists to provide educational information anyone can use to understand how herbs and botanical medicines play a vital role in optimal health. From a stomachache to a life-threatening disease, even cancer, the plant kingdom has safe, effective phytonutrients and answers for healthy living.

Author and health pioneer Terry Lemerond brings his vast knowledge of plant medicines combined with cutting edge research from today's top scientists and doctors directly to consumers.

Each TTN Publishing, LLC book is crafted to provide the necessary basic information and recommendations for how botanicals can be used in practical ways to fight disease and improve the path to healthy living.

Education, information, scientific validation, and common sense are a part of every TTN Publishing endeavor. There are many books to come, so stay connected! With 80 percent of the world's population depending on plant medicines, you can join in the knowledge and wisdom available to meet your health goals.

## WELCOME TO TTN PUBLISHING!

We'd love to hear from you!
info@ttnpublishing.com
www.TTNPublishing.com

Would you like to be one of the first to know the latest updates on Terry's books?

- Learn more about his background and new
- books
- See photos, videos, and the latest news
- Listen to Terry's radio show and podcasts, including archived programs on a multitude of subjects
- Sign up for a free weekly email newsletter and educational webinar notices

It's all available at www.TerryTalksNutrition.com

Don't forget to connect at:
facebook.com/TerryTalksNutrition

Visit and follow Terry's author page on Amazon - amazon.com/author/terrylemerond

## SHARE THIS EXCITING NEWS!

If you appreciated this book, please let others know.

- Pick up another copy and share with a friend
- Talk about it on social media
- Write a review on your blog or website
- Recommend this book to friends and family

Thank you for being a true health seeker!
**TTN Publishing, LLC**

## Also by Terry Lemerond and available on Amazon

(Free in Kindle Unlimited and available in eBook and paperback)

***Fight Disease with a Powerful, Natural Seed – The Wonders of French Grape Seed Extract***
*Prevent and Reverse: Cancer, Heart Disease, Diabetes, Alzheimer's & More*
by Terry Lemerond and Ajay Goel M.S. Ph.D.
https://www.amazon.com/Fight-Disease-Powerful-Natural-Seed-ebook/dp/B08MB12PF9

***Andrographis: The Natural Answer to Disease***
*Protection Against: Colds, flu, & upper respiratory infections, joint pain and arthritis, diabetes, heart disease, liver disease, cancer, and much more!*
by Terry Lemerond and Alexander Panossian, Ph.D.
https://www.amazon.com/ANDROGRAPHIS-NATURAL-DISEASE-Terry-Lemerond-ebook/dp/B08T9XS846

***Type 2 Diabetes?***
*Break Free Naturally with Hintonia*
by Terry Lemerond and Jacob Teitelbaum, M.D.
https://www.amazon.com/Type-Diabetes-Break-Naturally-Hintonia-ebook/dp/B08ZT3TVP4

***Relieve Pain Without Side Effects:***
*You Can Be Pain-free, Naturally!*
by Terry Lemerond and Jan McBarron M.D.
https://www.amazon.com/Relieve-Pain-Without-Side-Effects-ebook/dp/B091QCJW51

***Wake UP!***
*Melatonin is For More Than Just Sleep*
by Terry Lemerond and a forward by Jacob Teitelbaum, M.D
https://www.amazon.com/Wake-Melatonin-More-Than-Sleep-ebook/dp/B092KZHR88

***Trauma Comfrey, Nature's Healing Herb***
by Terry Lemerond and Holly Lucille, ND, RN
https://www.amazon.com/Trauma-Comfrey-Natures-Healing-Herb-ebook/dp/B09JWRMCLJ

***Drug-Free Relief of Anxiety & Stress***
by Terry Lemerond and Dr. Lynn Wagner
https://www.amazon.com/Drug-Free-Relief-Anxiety-Stress-Stress-Induced-ebook/dp/B09JWVQV18

***Propolis***
***The Natural Way to Prevent and Heal Infection:***
*Fights Infection Including: Bacterial, Viral, Fungal, Parasitic, and More*
by Terry Lemerond
https://www.amazon.com/Propolis-Natural-Prevent-Heal-Infection/dp/1952507227

***The Wise Ginseng Choice for Restored Health***
***HRG80™ Red Ginseng***
*The powerful answer to:*

- *Lack of Energy, Fatigue, Exhaustion*
- *Cancer, Diabetes, Alzheimer's and more*
- *Sexual Performance*

by Terry Lemerond and Jacob Teitelbaum, M.D.

Also available in paperback on Amazon:

***50+ Natural Health Secrets***
***Proven to Change Your Life***
by Terry Lemerond

Made in the USA
Monee, IL
05 November 2026

67962919R00052